Level 2

BTEC HEALTH AND SOCIAL CARE

ASSESSMENT GUIDE

Unit 6 THE IMPACT OF NUTRITION ON HEALTH AND WELLBEING

ELIZABETH RASHEED

HODDER EDUCATION
AN HACHETTE UK COMPANY

The sample learner answers provided in this assessment guide are intended to give guidance on how a learner might approach generating evidence for each assessment criterion. Answers do not necessarily include all of the evidence required to meet each assessment criterion. Assessor comments intend to highlight how sample answers might be improved to help learners meet the requirements of the grading criterion but are provided as a guide only. Sample answers and assessor guidance have not been verified by Edexcel and any information provided in this guide should not replace your own internal verification process.

Any work submitted as evidence for assessment for this unit must be the learner's own. Submitting as evidence, in whole or in part, any material taken from this guide will be regarded as plagiarism. Hodder Education accepts no responsibility for learners plagiarising work from this guide that does or does not meet the assessment criteria.

The sample assignment briefs are provided as a guide to how you might assess the evidence required for all or part of the internal assessment of this Unit. They have not been verified or endorsed by Edexcel and should be internally verified through your own Lead Internal Verifier as with any other assignment briefs, and/or checked through the BTEC assignment checking service.

Orders: please contact Bookpoint Ltd, 130 Milton Park, Abingdon, Oxon OX14 4SB. Telephone: +44 (0)1235 827720. Fax: +44 (0)1235 400454. Lines are open from 9.00 a.m. to 5.00 p.m., Monday to Saturday, with a 24-hour message answering service. You can also order through our website www.hoddereducation.co.uk

If you have any comments to make about this, or any of our other titles, please send them to educationenquiries@hodder.co.uk

British Library Cataloguing in Publication Data

A catalogue record for this title is available from the British Library

ISBN: 978 1 444 1 8980 3

Published 2013

Impression number 10 9 8 7 6 5 4 3 2 1

Year 2016 2015 2014 2013

Cover photo © RTimages – Fotolia.com

Typeset by Integra Software Services Pvt. Ltd., Pondicherry, India.

Printed in Dubai for Hodder Education,
an Hachette UK Company,
338 Euston Road,
London NW1 3BH

Contents

For the attention of the learner

You are not allowed to copy any information from this book and use it as your own evidence. That would count as plagiarism, which is taken very seriously and may result in disqualification. If you are in any doubt at all please speak to your teacher.

Acknowledgments

Photo credits

The authors and publishers would like to thank the following for permission to reproduce material in this book:

Page 3 (top) © a4stockphotos – Fotolia.com; (bottom) © Owen Price 2007 – iStockphoto.com; page 4 (top) © Morgan Lane Photography - iStockphoto.com; (bottom) © © Igor Dutina – Fotolia.com; page 5 (left) © volff – Fotolia.com; (right) © Julián Rovagnati – Fotolia.com; page 6 © Ingram Publishing Limited / Food Gold Vol 1 CD 3; page 9 © Stockbyte/ Getty Images Ltd/ Fast Food SD175; page 23 © Gogglebox / Alamy; page 24 © Lifescenes / Alamy.

Every effort has been made to trace and acknowledge ownership of copyright. The publishers will be happy to make suitable arrangements with any copyright holders whom it has not been possible to contact.

Command words

You will find the following command words in the assessment criteria for each unit.

Analyse	Identify the factors that apply and state how these are related. Explain the importance of each one.
Assess	Give careful consideration to all the factors or events that apply and identify which are the most important or relevant.
Compare	Identify the main factors that apply in two or more situations and explain the similarities and differences.
Create	Make or draw up a plan in order to meet the aims provided.
Describe	Give a clear description that includes all the relevant features – think of it as 'painting a picture with words'.
Discuss	Consider different aspects of a topic and how they interrelate, and the extent to which they are important.
Evaluate	Bring together all the information and review it to form a conclusion. Give evidence for each of your views or statements.
Explain	Provide details and give reasons and/or evidence to support the arguments being made. Start by introducing the topic then give the 'how' or 'why'.
Summarise	Demonstrate an understanding of the key facts, and if possible illustrate with relevant examples.

UNIT 6
The Impact of Nutrition on Health and Wellbeing

Unit 6: The Impact of Nutrition on Health and Wellbeing is an internally assessed, optional, specialist unit with two learning aims:

- Learning aim A: Explore the effects of balanced and unbalanced diets on the health and wellbeing of individuals.
- Learning aim B: Understand the specific nutritional needs and preferences of individuals.

The unit focuses on diet and its impact on health and wellbeing and starts by looking at the benefits of a balanced diet in aiding concentration and helping the body fight infection. Nutritional requirements vary with different life stages and different health needs. When this is understood, you will be able to make nutritional plans for individuals with specific requirements and you will be able to plan your own nutrition to improve your health and wellbeing.

Learning aim A looks at what makes up a balanced diet, and the effect that balanced diets and unbalanced diets have on individuals.

Learning aim B looks at understanding the specific nutritional needs and preferences of individuals. These needs vary for many reasons, and nutritional needs also vary with life stage. These variations must be considered when planning nutrition. By considering these factors in planning nutrition you will be preparing for a useful role in health and social care.

Each learning aim is divided into two sections. The first section focuses on the content of the learning aim and each of the topics are covered. At the end of each section there are some knowledge recap questions to test your understanding of the subject. The answers for the knowledge recap questions can be found at the end of the guide.

The second section of each learning aim provides support with assessment by using evidence generated by a student, for each grading criterion, with feedback from an assessor. The assessor has highlighted where the evidence is sufficient to satisfy the grading criterion and provided developmental feedback when additional work is required.

At the end of the guide are examples of assignment briefs for this unit. There is a sample assignment for each learning aim, and the tasks allow you to generate the evidence needed to meet all the assessment criteria in the unit.

Learning aim A

Explore the effects of balanced and unbalanced diets on the health and wellbeing of individuals

Assessment criteria

2A.P1 Describe the components of a balanced diet and their functions, sources and effects.

2A.P2 Describe the effects of an unbalanced diet on the health and wellbeing of individuals, giving examples of their causes.

2A.M1 Compare the effects of balanced and unbalanced diets on the health and wellbeing of two individuals.

2A.D1 Assess the long-term effects of a balanced and unbalanced diet on the health and wellbeing of individuals.

Dietary intake and food groups

This section looks at the components that make up a balanced diet, basic sources of nutrition and the function and effects of each component.

Essential nutrients

Studied

Essential nutrients are:

- carbohydrates: both simple (sugars), and complex (starch and non-starch polysaccharides (fibre))
- proteins: animal and plant sources
- fats and oils: animal fats, vegetable oils, fish oils
- vitamins: A, B (complex), C, D, E and K
- minerals: calcium, iron, sodium
- water.

Nutrients can be split into two groups. **Macro nutrients** are needed in the body in large amounts. These are proteins, fats and carbohydrates. **Micro nutrients** such as vitamins and minerals are needed in small amounts in our body.

Sources of nutrients

Studied

Nutrients can be found in the five food groups:

- meat, fish and meat and fish alternatives (such as tofu) provide protein (in the form of amino acids), some fats and oils and minerals such as sodium and iron
- fruit and vegetables provide many vitamins, especially vitamin C, fibre and some carbohydrates
- bread, other cereals and potatoes provide complex carbohydrates
- milk and dairy foods provide fats, some oils, vitamins A, B and D and calcium
- cakes and sweets provide sugars, or simple carbohydrates.

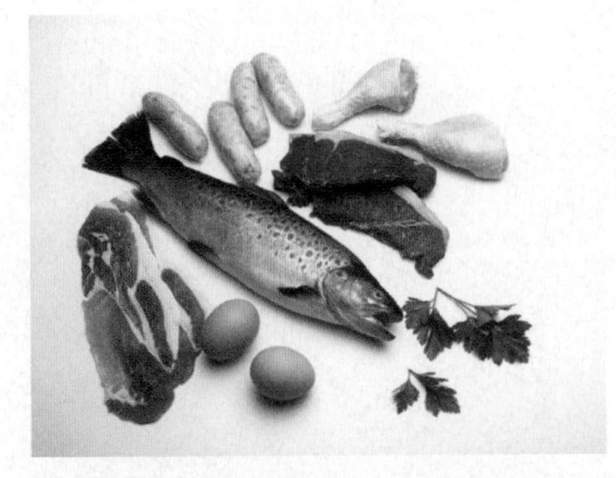

Figure 1.1 Meat and fish provide protein

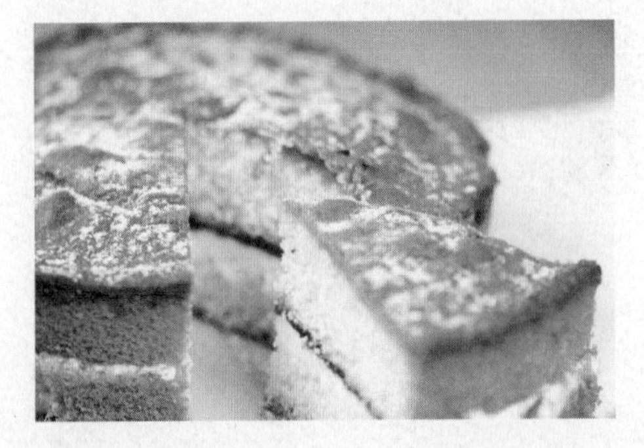

Figure 1.2 Cakes and sweets provide sugars and simple carbohydrates

The functions of food groups

Studied

The functions of food groups include growth, energy, and maintaining body functions.

Carbohydrates

Carbohydrates provide energy. Over half of the energy in our diets should come from carbohydrates. Sugar causes tooth decay therefore starch carbohydrates are better for you.

Non-starch polysaccharide is fibrous and our bodies cannot digest it, but it adds bulk to the diet, helps to prevent constipation and may prevent some bowel diseases.

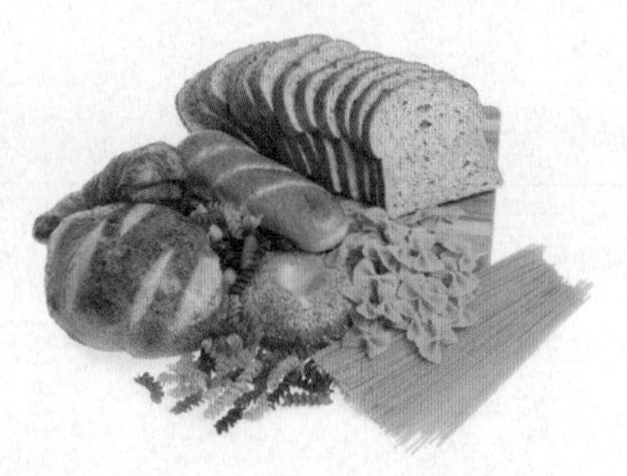

Figure 1.3 Bread and other cereals can be a source of complex carbohydrates

Proteins

Proteins repair new cells and help them grow. They build strong bones and teeth. The immune system, which fights infection, is made up of protein so babies, children, growing teenagers, older people and people who are ill, in particular, need a good supply of protein in their diets. Vegetarians and vegans (who do not eat meat or fish or dairy products) get protein from nuts, pulses (peas, beans and lentils), soya protein and some vegetables.

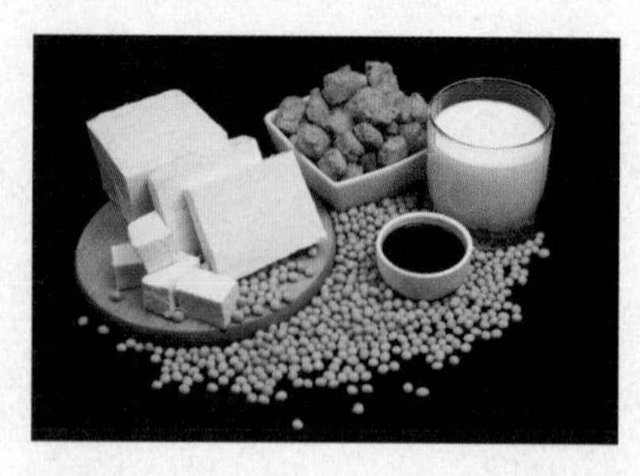

Figure 1.4 Foodstuffs like soya and tofu are a source of protein for vegetarians and vegans

Fats

Fat helps to protect vital organs in the body and also build cells. It provides energy and helps with the absorption of vitamins A, D, E and K into the body. Fat also provides taste and texture to food.

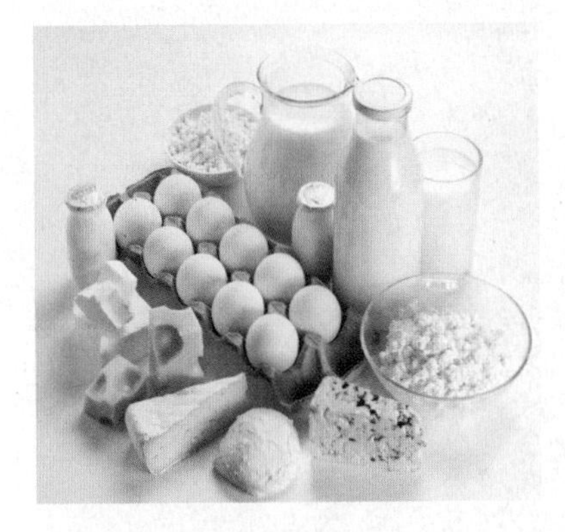

Figure 1.5 Milk and dairy products provide fats and protein

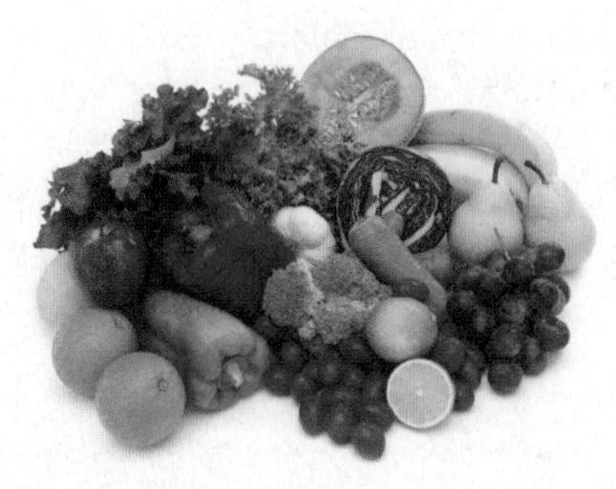

Figure 1.6 Fruits and vegetables provide many vitamins

Vitamins and minerals

Vitamins and minerals help maintain body functions. Different vitamins have different functions:

- Vitamin A – for vision in dim light, keeps skin healthy and mucous membranes (such as eyes and throat) free from infection, helps the growth of bones and teeth and helps fight infection.
- Vitamin B (complex) – helps utilise food energy, helps the body form red blood cells.
- Vitamin C – helps the absorption of iron and helps build bones and teeth, is needed for healthy skin and digestive system, helps fight infection by protecting the immune system.
- Vitamin D – for bones and teeth, helps the absorption of calcium.
- Vitamin E – an antioxidant, protects cells from damage, maintains a healthy reproductive system, nerves and muscles.
- Vitamin K – essential for blood clotting.
- Folate (Folic acid) – Particularly important for pregnant women as it helps the development of the baby's spinal cord.

Different minerals also have different functions:

- Calcium – makes strong teeth and bones; and helps with blood clotting and nerve functioning.
- Iron – carries oxygen in the blood to all cells.
- Sodium – keeps the fluid in the body in balance and is important for nerve and muscle impulses.
- Zinc – helps the immune system to function.

Water

Water makes up about 70 per cent of our body weight and has the following functions:

- regulating body temperature
- transporting nutrients
- enabling chemical reactions to take place
- maintaining bowel function.

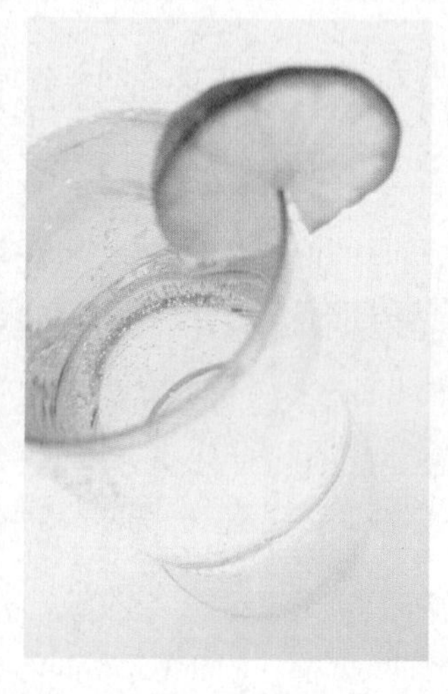

Figure 1.7 Water has many useful functions in the body

Recommended Daily Intakes

Studied

Recommended Daily Intakes (RDIs) are government guidelines for key nutrients.

Nutrient	1–3yrs	4–6yrs	7–10yrs	11–14yrs	15–18yrs	Adults 19–50 years	Adults 50 years +
Protein	15g	20g	28g	42g	55g	55g	53g
Iron	7mg	6mg	9mg	14.8mg	14.8mg	14.8mg	9mg
Zinc	5mg	6.5mg	7mg	9mg	9.5mg	9.5mg	9.5mg
Vitamin A	400mcg	400mcg	500mcg	600mcg	700mcg	700mcg	700mcg
Folate	70mcg	100mcg	150mcg	200mcg	200mcg	200mcg	200mcg
Vitamin C	30mg	30mg	30mg	35mg	40mg	40mg	40mg
Salt (sodium)	2g	3g	5g	6g	6g	6g	6g

Table 1.1 FSA nutrient and food-based guidelines for UK institutions (revised October 2007). Source: Food Standards Agency

Long-term effects of balanced and unbalanced diets

Effects of a balanced diet

Studied

The effects of a balanced diet include:

- raised immunity to infections – better ability to fight off infections
- greater energy levels and increased concentration
- faster healing of skin, tissues and mucus membranes.

The effects of an unbalanced diet

Studied

The effects of an unbalanced diet include:

- malnutrition
- vitamin deficiency
- mineral deficiency
- nutrient excess.

Malnutrition

This can be malnutrition due to the intake of too many nutrients or too few:

Over-nutrition – eating too much. Causes coronary heart disease, which can cause heart attacks or heart failure, also obesity, type 2 diabetes, stroke and weight gain.

Under-nutrition – eating too little of the right nutrients, causes nutrient deficiency diseases. A shortage of calcium can lead to rickets, where bones are soft and leg bones may curve as they are not strong enough to bear the weight of the body. Under-nutrition also causes a low concentration span. Vegetarians/vegans who do not eat meat, fish or dairy foods are at risk of protein, vitamin and mineral deficiency, so must take care to eat lentils, pulses, nuts and seeds to get these nutrients.

Vitamin deficiency

Vitamin	Found in	Shortage leads to
A (Retinol)	Animal foods, milk, cheese, eggs, oily fish, fruit and vegetables	Poor vision in dim light, low resistance to infections and accelerated ageing.
B1 – Thiamin	Milk, eggs, vegetables, fruit	Beriberi (where a person is very weak), depression and problems with the nervous system.
B2 – Riboflavin	Milk and milk products	Sore mouth and tongue.
B3 – Niacin	Cheese, meat (especially chicken)	Skin peeling, diarrhoea, memory loss, insomnia.
B6 – Pyridoxine	Meat, fish, eggs	Nerve problems and fatigue.
B12 – Cyanocobalamin	Meat (especially liver), milk, eggs, cheese	Pernicious anaemia and degeneration of nerve cells.
Folate (Folic acid)	Leafy green vegetables, potatoes and oranges	Anaemia.
C (Ascorbic acid)	Fresh fruit, vegetables and fruit juices	Cracks at the corner of the mouth, scurvy and poor healing of wounds.
D (Cholecalciferol)	Found in fish liver oils, oily fish, eggs, dairy products, and margarine. Also produced by exposure to sunlight	Weak bones and teeth. Bones bend, causing rickets in children, bone loss (osteoporosis), low blood calcium, brittle bones, and impaired tooth formation.
E (Tocopherol)	Vegetable oils, nuts and egg yolk	Lethargy, apathy, muscle weakness.
K	In many foods, including leafy vegetables such as spinach and cauliflower	Bleeding, as blood does not clot.

Mineral deficiency

Mineral	Sources	Effect of shortage
Calcium	Milk, cheese, eggs, bones of canned fish. It is also added to white flour by law	Poor teeth development, rickets in children and osteomalacia in adults. Tetany (lockjaw) may result if muscles and nerves do not function properly.
Iron	Red meat, offal, fish, dark leafy green vegetables, pulses, cereal, nuts, dried herbs and spices	Shortage causes anaemia, particularly in infants 6–12 months, teenage girls who are menstruating and older people.
Sodium	Found in many additives, snacks and preservatives, naturally found in eggs, meat and vegetables	Shortage causes muscle cramps.

Nutrient excess

Nutrient excess can cause problems too:

- Too much fat in the diet (for example, too many chips) can lead to obesity and heart failure.
- Too much simple carbohydrate in the form of sugar (for example, in fizzy drinks) causes tooth decay, obesity and can lead to mood swings.
- Too much vitamin A can be toxic as the liver cannot process it.
- Too much sodium causes high blood pressure, which can lead to a stroke.

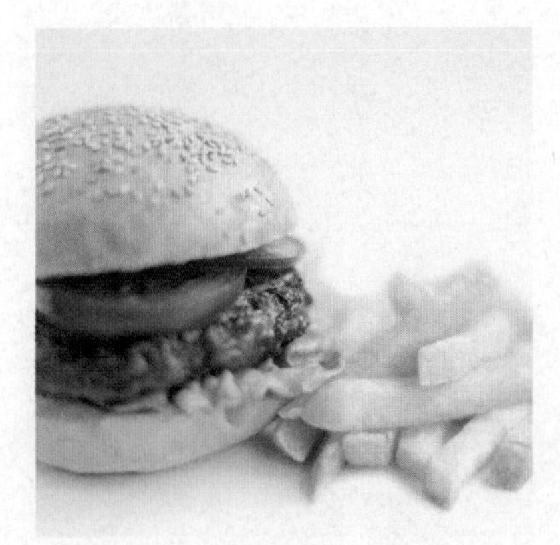

Figure 1.8 Too many chips and other fatty products can lead to obesity and heart disease

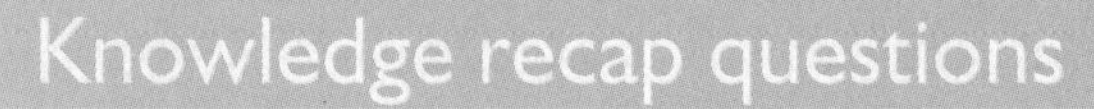

Knowledge recap questions

1. Name the five main food groups.
2. What is the main function of each of these food groups?
3. Name the vitamin that gives better night vision.
4. Which vitamin helps blood to clot?
5. Which mineral is needed to prevent anaemia?

Assessment guidance for Learning aim A

Scenario

As part of your voluntary work at a health centre you have been asked to present information to the service users about components of a balanced diet, its functions and sources, and explain and analyse the potential effects of healthy and unhealthy diets on their health and wellbeing. You could present your work as a leaflet, booklet or poster.

2A.P1 Describe the components of a balanced diet and their functions, sources and effects.

Assessor report: The command verb in the grading criteria is **describe**. We would expect to see a description of the components of a balanced diet, for example carbohydrates, their functions, sources (e.g. bread, pasta) and their main effects.

Learner answer

Component	Function	Source	Effects
Carbohydrates – both simple (sugars), and complex (starch and fibre)	They give energy.	Sugars – sweets, fizzy drinks Starch – potatoes, bread, rice, pasta	Sugars give a quick boost of energy. Starch releases energy slowly and keeps us from feeling hungry.
Proteins	They repair and help new cells grow such as muscles.	Meat, fish, eggs, lentils, peas and beans	Protein helps the body grow and develop.
Fats and oils	They protect the nerves and organs such as the kidneys, help with absorption of vitamins A, D, E and K and also store extra energy.	Animal fats such as butter or margarine, vegetable oils, fish oils	We need some fat to maintain the body and give us energy. Fat helps our nervous system work properly.
Vitamins A, B (complex), C, D, E and K			

Minerals: calcium, iron, sodium			
Water	Regulates body temperature, carries nutrients, enables digestion to take place.	Tap water, fruit juice	Keeps the body in balance. Gets rid of impurities and helps prevent constipation.

Assessor report: The learner has listed each of the components of a balance diet and has described some of the components of a balanced diet, their functions, sources and effects.

Assessor report – overall

What is good about this assessment evidence?

The learner has presented work in a clearly laid out table and has researched information from a range of sources.

What could be improved about this assessment evidence?

In order to achieve 2A.P1, the learner should describe the functions, sources and effects of vitamins and minerals. It would be a good idea to have a separate line for each of the vitamins A, B (complex), C, D, E and K and to have a separate line for each of the three minerals.

2A.P2 Describe the effects of an unbalanced diet on the health and wellbeing of individuals, giving examples of their causes.

Assessor report: The command verb in the grading criteria is **describe**. In the learner's answer we would expect to see details of the effects of an unbalanced diet, and examples of their causes. At least three effects of an unbalanced diet on the health and wellbeing of individuals are needed. This could be included on the leaflet.

Learner answer

An unbalanced diet can have too much of one component or not enough of a component. The effects of an unbalanced diet are:

- being overweight or underweight
- a lack of energy
- always getting colds and having no resistance to infections.

Effect of an unbalanced diet	Cause
Mood swings, tiredness, thirst, tooth decay	Too much sugar in the diet
Being overweight, breathless when walking, spotty skin	Too much fat and or carbohydrate
Spotty skin, poor healing of cuts, mouth ulcers	Lack of vitamin C

Assessor report: The learner has made a good start in identifying some of the effects of an unbalanced diet.

Assessor report – overall

What is good about this assessment evidence?

The learner has set out the table with clear headings and identified three effects of an unbalanced diet.

What could be improved about this assessment evidence?

The learner has identified effects of an unbalanced diet but needs to add more detail to provide a description, for example that too much sugar in the diet can cause mood swings, so a child who drinks a lot of cola and eats a lot of sweets could be excitable and overactive when they consume sugary drinks and sweets and later feel tired and irritable. The learner should describe malnutrition, vitamin deficiency and mineral deficiency as well as nutrient excess.

2A.M1 Compare the effects of balanced and unbalanced diets on the health and wellbeing of two individuals.

Assessor report: The command verb in the grading criteria is compare. The learner's answer should include case studies that allow them to compare the effects of balanced and unbalanced diets on the health and wellbeing of two individuals. This would be a balanced and also an unbalanced diet for individual one, then a balanced and unbalanced diet for individual two.

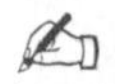 **Learner answer**

Case study A: A sixteen-year-old boy who plays active sports three times a week

A balanced diet

A balanced diet for this individual would be based around slow-release energy foods which are carbohydrates. Proteins are needed as a sixteen-year-old is still growing and needs muscle-building protein. Vitamins are needed to promote healing of cuts and bruises. Minerals are needed; for example, iron to prevent anaemia, calcium to strengthen bone.

A balanced diet will include slow-release carbohydrates such as pasta, boiled or jacket potatoes and rice to give energy. Wholemeal and wholegrain bread will give vitamins, iron and minerals as well as providing fibre to keep the gut healthy.

Protein in the form of chicken and fish will build and repair cells without adding too much fat. Chicken also provides iron and sodium. Fruit such as oranges will give vitamin C and green leafy vegetables will provide vitamins A for improved vision, C for improved wound healing, and K to help blood clot and heal wounds.

Minerals such as calcium, some fat and vitamins A and D are in milk. This is also a good source of protein to repair cells.

Water is an essential part of a balanced diet as it helps the body use food efficiently and also keeps the gut healthy.

The effects of a balanced diet are that the person is the right weight, has energy, resists infections and when they do have an injury, their body heals quickly.

An unbalanced diet

An unbalanced diet may lead to malnutrition, vitamin deficiency, mineral deficiency, as well as nutrient excess.

In an unbalanced diet, with nutrient excess, there is likely to be an excess of carbohydrates and fats in the form of chips, which are starch cooked in fat. Sugary drinks provide a quick energy boost but cause dehydration and tooth decay. White bread has fewer nutrients and may cause bowel problems. Pastry, for example, in pies and pasties provides further carbohydrates with fats. Fat is also found in chips, burgers, and pies, fried eggs and bacon, and fried steak. The effect of a diet high in fats and carbohydrates is likely to be obesity, lack of energy, and tiredness.

Fatty foods and carbohydrates give a full feeling so protein intake may be lower in an unbalanced diet. The body is slow to repair any damage. If there are not enough fresh fruits or vegetables in the diet there is likely to be vitamin deficiency so resistance to infection is low and wounds take longer to heal.

Mineral deficiency occurs in an unbalanced diet. Lack of calcium causes weak bones that fracture easily. Lack of iron causes anaemia and breathlessness. Lack of sodium causes muscle cramps. The effect is that it is difficult for the person to be fit and to keep healthy. This is an example of malnourishment with nutrient excess. Sometimes people just do not eat enough of anything and are malnourished with all-round nutrient deficiency, which causes tiredness and lack of energy.

Comparing the effects of a balanced diet and an unbalanced diet for a sixteen-year-old boy who plays sports, we can see that the balanced diet gives him the best chance of being healthy and being able to maintain his fitness for sport. It provides a steady supply of energy, protein and vitamins to heal wounds quickly, and maintains him at a healthy weight .A diet unbalanced in fat will encourage obesity which will make it difficult for him to be active. Sugary carbohydrates will burn quickly, leaving him exhausted. He will be prone to infections as he lacks vitamins, and his bones will be weak due to lack of calcium **(a)**.

Assessor report: The learner has made a good start in describing and comparing a balanced and an unbalanced diet for a specific individual.

Assessor report – overall

What is good about this assessment evidence?

The learner has considered the effects of each of these diets on the health and wellbeing of one individual. They have compared the effects of each diet on the health and wellbeing of that individual **(a)**.

What could be improved about this assessment evidence?

In order to achieve 2A.M1, the learner needs do the same with a different case study, choosing someone of a different age to draw out the differing dietary needs.

2A.D1 Assess the long-term effects of a balanced and unbalanced diet on the health and wellbeing of individuals.

Assessor report: The command verb in the grading criteria is **assess**, and the focus is on long-term effects. The learner can build on their work for 2A.M1 and add the long-term effects of having a balanced or an unbalanced diet and an assessment of these effects.

Learner answer

Case study A: A sixteen-year-old boy who plays active sports three times a week

A balanced diet

A balanced diet would be based around slow-release energy foods which are carbohydrates. Proteins are needed as a sixteen-year-old is still growing and needs muscle-building protein. Vitamins are needed to promote healing of cuts and bruises. Minerals are needed; for example, iron to prevent anaemia, calcium to strengthen bone.

A balanced diet will include slow-release carbohydrates such as pasta, boiled or jacket potatoes and rice to give energy. Wholemeal and wholegrain bread will give vitamins, iron and minerals as well as providing fibre to keep the gut healthy.

Protein in the form of chicken and fish will build and repair cells without adding too much fat. Chicken also provides iron and sodium. Fruit such as oranges will give vitamin C and green leafy vegetables will provide vitamins A for improved vision, C for improved wound healing, and K to help blood clot and heal wounds.

Minerals such as calcium, some fat and vitamins A and D are in milk. This is also a good source of protein to repair cells.

Water is an essential part of a balanced diet as it helps the body use food efficiently and also keeps the gut healthy.

The effects of a balanced diet are that the person is the right weight, has energy, resists infections and when they do have an injury, their body heals quickly.

An unbalanced diet

An unbalanced diet may lead to malnutrition, vitamin deficiency, mineral deficiency, as well as nutrient excess.

In an unbalanced diet, with nutrient excess, there is likely to be an excess of carbohydrates and fats in the form of chips, which are starch cooked in fat. Sugary drinks provide a quick energy boost but cause dehydration and tooth decay. White bread has fewer nutrients and may cause bowel problems. Pastry, for example, in pies and pasties, provides further carbohydrates with fats. Fat is also found in chips, burgers, and pies, fried eggs and bacon, and fried steak. The effect of a diet high in fats and carbohydrates is likely to be obesity, lack of energy and tiredness.

Fatty foods and carbohydrates give a full feeling so protein intake may be lower in an unbalanced diet. The body is slow to repair any damage. If there are not enough fresh fruits or vegetables in the diet there is likely to be vitamin deficiency so resistance to infection is low and wounds take longer to heal.

Mineral deficiency occurs in an unbalanced diet. Lack of calcium causes weak bones that fracture easily. Lack of iron causes anaemia and breathlessness. Lack of sodium causes muscle cramps. The effect is that it is difficult for the person to be fit and to keep healthy. This is an example of malnourishment with nutrient excess.

Sometimes people just do not eat enough of anything and are malnourished with all-round nutrient deficiency which causes tiredness and lack of energy.

Comparing the effects of a balanced diet and an unbalanced diet for a sixteen-year-old boy who plays sports, we can see that the balanced diet gives him the best chance of being healthy and being able to maintain his fitness for sport. It provides a steady supply of energy, protein and vitamins to heal wounds quickly, and maintains him at a healthy weight. A diet unbalanced in fat will encourage obesity which will make it difficult for him to be active. Sugary carbohydrates will burn quickly, leaving him exhausted. He will be prone to infections as he lacks vitamins, and his bones will be weak due to lack of calcium.

Assessing the long-term effects of a balanced and unbalanced diet on the health and wellbeing of the sixteen-year-old boy

The balanced diet will enable the boy to maintain his weight and fitness levels so he can continue with sport for many years. This will, in turn, strengthen muscles and bones, keep the circulation healthy and prevent the build up of fat in the body. It is likely that his lungs and heart will be healthy and that he will live to a healthy old age.

An unbalanced diet will, however, lead to problems in the long term. Coronary heart disease, obesity, type 2 diabetes and stroke are likely to be the long-term effect of an unbalanced diet. Obesity is the first effect, when too many calories are taken in and stored in the body as fat.

Fatty deposits block the arteries supplying the heart, and cause pain known as angina. When fat deposits break off they can block arteries supplying the brain and cause a stroke. Type 2 diabetes occurs mainly in people who have excessive amounts of high-sugar foods and drinks, processed foods and high-fat foods over a long time.

The pancreas stops working, insulin is not produced and glucose stays in the blood stream eventually damaging blood vessels, nerves and organs. The long-term effects of an unbalanced diet are likely to be either disability, for example, being paralysed after a stroke, or the effects may be early death due to a heart attack.

Assessor report: The learner has made a good start in assessing the long-term effects of a balanced and unbalanced diet on the health and wellbeing of one individual.

Assessor report – overall

What is good about this assessment evidence?

The learner has given specific detail of the long-term effects of each diet, making an assessment of these effects.

What could be improved about this assessment evidence?

To achieve 2A.D1, the learner should do the same with a different case study, choosing someone of a different age and drawing out the long-term effects of a balanced and unbalanced diet on the health and wellbeing of the second individual.

Learning aim B

Understand the specific nutritional needs and preferences of individuals

Assessment criteria

2B.P3 Describe the specific dietary needs of two individuals at different life stages.

2B.M2 Explain the factors influencing the dietary choices of two individuals with specific dietary needs at different life stages.

2B.D2 Discuss how factors influence the dietary choices of two individuals with specific dietary needs at different life stages.

2B.P4 Create a nutritional plan for two individuals with different specific nutritional needs.

2B.M3 Compare nutritional plans for two individuals with different nutritional needs.

Factors influencing the diet of individuals and their associated dietary needs

Several factors influence the dietary needs of individuals but it never safe to make assumptions about what an individual wants to eat. Always ask the person.

Religion and culture

Studied

Religious or cultural beliefs can affect what a person does or does not eat. For example:

- **Hinduism** – Hindus do not eat meat, fish or eggs. Alcohol is forbidden.
- **Judaism** – Jews eat kosher food. Meat must be prepared in a ritually acceptable manner. Meat and dairy products are not eaten in the same meal and pork is forbidden.

- **Islam** – Believers in Islam are Muslims. Meat must be prepared in a ritually acceptable manner (halal). Pork is forbidden. Alcohol is forbidden.
- **Buddhism** – Many Buddhists are vegetarian. They do not drink alcohol. Buddhists avoid strong foods such as onions and garlic.

Moral reasons

Studied

Vegans eat a plant-based diet and therefore they avoid foods like meat, fish, milk, eggs and honey. A vegetarian will avoid meat and fish products.

Environment

Studied

Environment or location influences diet. In this country, large supermarkets are usually on out-of-town sites and transport is needed to access them. Those without transport cannot get to these stores. People who live close to shops and can afford to shop will be able to have enough food and a choice of food. Those who do not live near shops may have to survive on what they produce. In many parts of the world, if crops fail due to drought or flood, people may starve, or if there is a good harvest and no means of storing food, the food will rot.

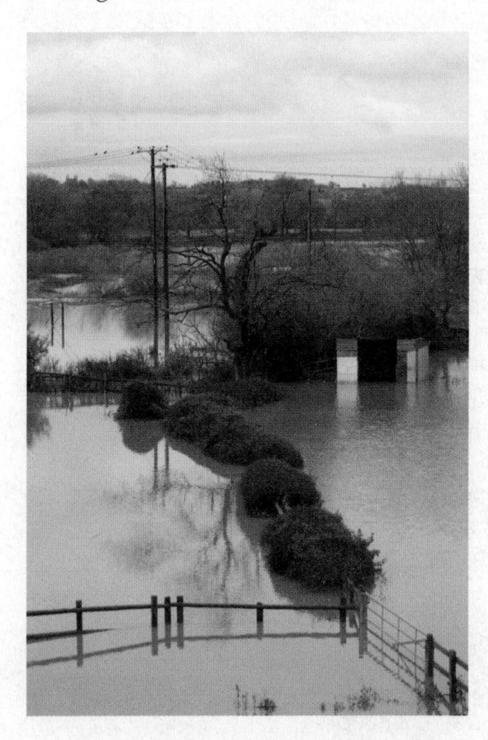

Figure 2.1 Crops may fail due to drought or flood

Socio-economic factors

Studied

People on a limited budget may have less choice in their diet. Different social classes make different dietary choices. Those from higher social classes may eat a healthier diet because they are educated and can afford better food, whereas people from a lower social class with less money may not be able to afford it, or may not know which foods are healthy. People around you can also influence your dietary choices. Television, magazines, leaflets, posters, published research articles and news events (i.e. 'The Media') influence our food choices. Fast-food companies target young people showing fast-food outlets as a place to meet friends and eat at a price they can afford.

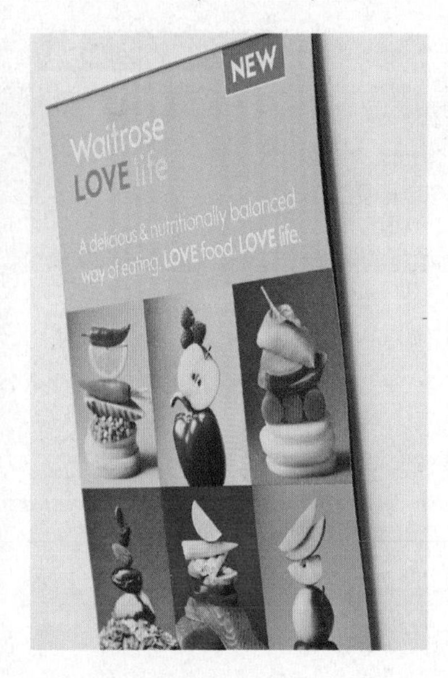

Figure 2.2 Our food choices are affected by many outside influences

The position in the family may determine your dietary choices. Women sometimes eat poorer quality food when money is scarce, giving the best food to their children.

Personal preferences

Studied

Some people dislike certain foods. Within one family someone may refuse to eat fish while another person loves it. Some may not have breakfast while others do.

Illness

Studied

When people are ill, they often eat less than usual. If this reduced food intake continues for a long time, it can cause weight loss, malnutrition and death. People with illnesses should be encouraged to follow good eating habits, including high-protein and high-energy foods. Fruits with vitamin C will aid healing.

Underlying health condition resulting in specific nutritional needs

Studied

Underlying health condition	Diet required
Food allergies	
An allergy is a reaction of the body to an allergen. Allergens can include foods, such as nuts, fruits, dairy products and gluten in wheat.	Avoid the known allergen. Always check labels on packaging.
Lactose intolerance	
Lactose is a sugar present in dairy products. Some people are unable to digest this sugar in their diet. It causes stomach cramps and diarrhoea.	Dairy products should be replaced with soya based foods, e.g. soya milk and non-dairy products.
Gluten/wheat allergy (coeliac disease)	
Gluten is present in wheat, barley and oats. Allergy to gluten affects the digestive system and prevents correct absorption of nutrients.	Replace foods that contain wheat, barley and oats with gluten-free products.
Diabetes	
Fluctuating sugar levels may cause sweating, thirst and coma.	The diet should contain measured amounts of carbohydrates that are low-glycaemic, which means glucose is produced from the foods gradually to maintain a constant energy level.
Irritable bowel syndrome (IBS)	
Can be caused by over-activity in the gut, which causes both constipation and diarrhoea. Situations of stress can make this condition worse.	Make time to relax. Some research recommends a high-fibre diet, which maintains regular bowel movements.
Crohn's disease	
No known cause for this disorder but it may be genetic and can be made worse by smoking, long-term antibiotics, and previous infections of the gut.	Certain foods, such as dairy products, fatty foods and spicy foods may worsen symptoms in some people. Identifying the triggers and eliminating them from the diet may help.

Nutritional variation during life stage development

Life stage	Dietary suggestions
Preconception and pregnancy	Before pregnancy, the couple should aim to both be in good health and should consider their diet and alcohol intake. High levels of alcohol can affect sperm production and in pregnancy can affect the child intellectually and physically. During pregnancy the woman should include folic acid in her balanced diet, which helps the development of the spinal cord in the baby. Protein is also essential for new growth. However foods that contain live bacteria should be avoided, for example unpasteurised milk, cheese and uncooked eggs.
Infancy (0–2 years)	Up until around 6 months old the baby should be totally breastfed or given formula milk, depending on the choice of the parents. Weaning onto solid foods is not recommended until after six months. Include a variety of tastes in a smooth consistency, gradually getting lumpier so the baby can learn to chew.
Early childhood (3–8 years)	The diet should be high in protein as the child is growing rapidly. Carbohydrates are required for energy, as the child is becoming more mobile and learning new skills. Calcium and vitamin D are required for bone and tooth development. Avoid sugary drinks and sweet food, and avoid additives in food.
Adolescence (9–18 years)	Girls reaching puberty need a diet high in iron. All adolescents require protein in their diets as growth spurts are common at this life stage. Peer pressure may lead to eating 'junk' foods, which can lead to obesity and tooth decay. Education is required about the benefits of a balanced diet and the dangers of excessive alcohol intake.
Early to middle adulthood (19–65 years)	Adults should have a balanced diet to supply enough calories to match the activity level of the person This requirement varies according to lifestyle and occupation. Builders may need more calories than office workers. Pregnant women may need iron supplements. Lactating women need a healthy diet and sufficient calories to produce milk. Later in adulthood the metabolism slows down so portion sizes should be adjusted.
Later adulthood (65 years +)	Activity often slows down so the diet should be lower in fats and contain more protein to help with repair of cells particularly in times of illness. The diet should contain calcium to help maintain bone density. Portion sizes should also be reduced if the person is less active.

Considerations for nutritional planning

This is a practical section where learners are expected to apply their knowledge of dietary intake, long-term effects of balanced and unbalanced diets, and specific nutritional needs and preferences to create nutritional plans for individuals.

Learners should consider the following for nutritional planning:

- Factors influencing the diet of individuals and their associated dietary needs (as listed above).
- The life stage of the individual and their associated nutritional requirements, e.g. in infancy, early childhood, adolescence, early and middle adulthood, later adulthood.

Knowledge recap questions

1. What factors influence dietary needs?
2. If someone has lactose intolerance, what must they avoid?
3. When should weaning start?
4. What two nutrients are very important for the growing young child?
5. In later adulthood, why should calcium be included in the diet?

Assessment guidance for Learning aim B

Scenario

The practice nurse now asks you to create a nutritional plan for two people, outlining their specific needs and considering their different life stages and specific dietary needs.

The nurse has asked you to use two case studies based on different age groups and different health needs, for example, a teenager with coeliac disease and a retired person with type 2 diabetes. You will need to describe their specific dietary needs, discuss factors influencing their dietary choices, such as cost, convenience, religion or personal preferences.

2B.P3 Describe the specific dietary needs of two individuals at different life stages.

Assessor report: The command verb in the grading criteria is describe. In the learner's answer we would expect to see a description of the specific dietary needs for two individuals.

Learner answer

Kaye is 15 years old and she wants to become a nurse. She likes swimming and going out with her friends. She has coeliac disease, which means that her body cannot process the gluten protein found in wheat, barley and rye. If she eats foods with gluten, the gluten causes an immune reaction, which damages the lining of her small intestine. Foods containing gluten are bread, pasta, breakfast cereals, flour, pizza bases, cakes and biscuits. Some soups, ready meals and processed foods such as sausages also contain gluten. This means she cannot go for a burger or a pizza as she gets bloating, wind and diarrhoea and a skin rash if she eats them. If she carries on eating foods with gluten, her small intestine may become so damaged that it will no longer absorb the nutrients from what she eats.

As a teenager, Kaye needs lots of protein as she is still growing, and she needs minerals such as iron, calcium, sodium and vitamins such as vitamin C to help her body heal. Gluten-free foods are meat, fish, fruit and vegetables, rice, potatoes and lentils. She can get protein from lentils, meat and fish, vitamins from fruit and vegetables, minerals from meat and fish, and she can also get energy from carbohydrates such as rice and potatoes.

Assessor report: The learner has made a good start in describing the dietary needs of one teenager with coeliac disease.

Assessor report – overall

What is good about this assessment evidence?

The learner has given details of the individual's dietary needs, stating what the disorder is, how the body reacts, what foods the individual must avoid and what she can have.

What could be improved about this assessment evidence?

To achieve 2B.P3, a second example is needed. The learner must make sure that their second individual is from a different age group and has differing dietary needs.

2B.M2 Explain the factors influencing the dietary choices of two individuals with specific dietary needs at different life stages.

Assessor report: The command verb in the grading criteria is **explain**. In the learner's answer we would expect to see development of the work they have completed for 2B.P3, explaining factors to be considered, for example access to food, budget, culture or religion.

Learner answer

Kaye is 15 years old, her mum is English and her dad is from Pakistan. She wants to become a nurse. She likes swimming and going out with her friends. She has coeliac disease, which means that her body cannot process the gluten protein found in wheat, barley and rye. If she eats foods with gluten, the gluten causes an immune reaction, which damages the lining of her small intestine. Foods containing gluten are bread, pasta, breakfast cereals, flour, pizza bases, cakes and biscuits. Some soups, ready meals and processed foods such as sausages also include gluten. This means she cannot go for a burger or a pizza as she gets bloating, wind and diarrhoea and a skin rash if she eats them. If she carries on eating foods with gluten, her small intestine may become so damaged that it will no longer absorb the nutrients from what she eats **(a)**.

As a teenager, Kaye needs lots of protein as she is still growing, and she needs minerals such as iron, calcium, sodium and vitamins such as vitamin C to help her body heal **(a)**. Gluten-free foods are meat, fish, fruit and vegetables, rice, potatoes and lentils. She can get protein from lentils, meat and fish, vitamins from fruit and vegetables, minerals from meat and fish, and she can also get energy from carbohydrates such as rice and potatoes.

Kaye's diet is influenced not only by her coeliac disease but also by other factors such as access to food, budget, culture or religion. Access to food **(b)** is an issue for Kaye because she is at school all day and the school canteen mostly serves soup, sandwiches, pizza, and pasta. Occasionally they have rice but it is usually with meat curry and is too expensive **(c)** for Kaye as the family do not have a lot of money and she does not like to ask her parents for too much since her dad was made redundant. She is also not able to eat curry the way they make it at school as they put flour (which contains gluten) in to thicken the sauce. She prefers a proper curry like her dad makes with onions to thicken the sauce **(d)**.

Assessor report: The learner has made a good start, explaining the factors influencing diet for one individual.

Assessor report – overall

What is good about this assessment evidence?

The learner has given specific examples of the factors affecting one individual's dietary choice, physical factors related to gluten intolerance **(a)**, access to food **(b)**, budgetary factors **(c)**, and cultural factors **(d)**.

What could be improved about this assessment evidence?

To achieve 2B.M2, a second case study is required from a different age group, with differing needs and with differing factors influencing dietary choice.

2B.D2 Discuss how factors influence the dietary choices of two individuals with specific dietary needs at different life stages.

Assessor report: The command verb in the grading criteria is discuss. In the learner's answer we would expect to see a consideration of the different effects of these factors on two individuals with specific dietary needs, for example how having little money reduces choice and how any difficulties may be overcome. Case studies, whether provided by the centre or written by the learner, should include enough detail about factors affecting individuals' specific dietary needs so that learners can use this information when considering diet.

*Distinction points are added in **bold** in this example.*

Learner answer

Kaye is 15 years old , her mum is English and her dad is from Pakistan. She wants to become a nurse. She likes swimming and going out with her friends. She has coeliac disease which means that her body cannot process the gluten protein found in wheat, barley and rye. If she eats foods with gluten, the gluten causes an immune reaction which damages the lining of her small intestine. Foods containing gluten are bread, pasta, breakfast cereals, flour, pizza bases, cakes and biscuits. Some soups, ready meals and processed foods such as sausages also include gluten. This means she cannot go for a burger or a pizza as she gets bloating, wind and diarrhoea and a skin rash if she eats them. If she carries on eating foods with gluten, her small intestine may become so damaged that it will no longer absorb the nutrients from what she eats.

As a teenager, Kaye needs lots of protein as she is still growing, and she needs minerals such as iron, calcium, sodium and vitamins such as vitamin C to help her body heal. Gluten-free foods are meat, fish, fruit and vegetables, rice, potatoes and lentils. She can get protein from lentils, meat and fish, vitamins from fruit and vegetables, minerals from meat and fish, and she can also get energy from carbohydrates such as rice and potatoes.

Kaye's diet is influenced not only by her coeliac disease but also by other factors such as access to food, budget, culture or religion. Access to food is an issue for Kaye because she is at school all day and the school canteen mostly serves soup, sandwiches, pizza, and pasta. Occasionally they have rice but it is usually with meat curry and is too expensive for Kaye as the family do not have a lot of money and she does not like to ask her parents for too much since her dad was made redundant. She is also not able to eat curry the way they make it at school as they put flour (which contains gluten) in to thicken the sauce. She prefers a proper curry like her dad makes with onions to thicken the sauce.

For Kaye, the most important factor influencing her choice of food has to be her gluten intolerance. If she ignores this and tries to eat whatever her friends are having, she will have unpleasant symptoms in the short term but in the long term she will cause serious damage to her body. This is not a factor she can overcome (a). Access to suitable food is, however, a problem that can be overcome (a). The choice of food she can eat is limited, so she takes a packed lunch every day. In this way she can have a varied diet that is gluten-free and gives her all the nutrients she needs. It is healthier as she can take a salad from home and have rice or potatoes and meat. Lack of money is a factor that she cannot do much about but she can overcome the difficulty it causes (a). She cannot afford to buy fruit or have a varied diet if she buys it in school but taking her own works out cheaper, thus overcoming the problem of not having money. The only difficulty she has is getting up a bit earlier to pack her lunch.

Assessor report: The learner has made a good start by discussing the factors influencing dietary choice and their relative importance **(a)** for one specific individual.

Assessor report –overall

What is good about this assessment evidence?

The learner gives specific examples for one individual of the effects of each factor and how difficulties could be overcome **(a)**. The learner also discussed the relative importance of these factors.

What could be improved about this assessment evidence?

To achieve 2B.D2, the learner needs to complete their answer by including the second case study and considering each of the factors indicated for 2B.P3, 2B.M2 and 2B.D2.

2B.P4 Create a nutritional plan for two individuals with different specific nutritional needs.

Assessor report: The command verb in the grading criteria is create. In the learner's answer we would expect to see a nutritional plan for two individuals with specific nutritional needs at different life stages, following on from 2B.P3. Here the focus is on application of knowledge and understanding of dietary intake, long-term effects of balanced and unbalanced diets, and the specific nutritional needs and preferences of the two individuals to create appropriate nutritional plans for the two individuals.

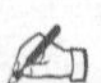 **Learner answer**

Nutritional plan for Kaye, a teenager with *coeliac disease*

The plan shows a balanced diet high in protein, vitamins and minerals, avoiding gluten. Kaye likes fruit and vegetables and likes curry, therefore the plan has been devised around her preferences. She also requires a packed lunch during the week, therefore lunches consist of salads and food that can be prepared the night before. She has high energy needs, therefore a diet of around 2000 calories may be needed, mostly from potatoes, rice and gluten-free cereals.

	Mon	Tue	Wed	Thu	Fri	Sat	Sun
B'FAST	A fresh orange, cup of milk, slice of gluten-free bread **(a)**	Skimmed milk, banana and small yoghurt	Gluten-free **(a)** cereal, skimmed milk, banana	Gluten-free **(a)** cereal, skimmed milk, grapefruit	Gluten-free **(a)** cereal, skimmed milk, apple	Blueberries and gluten-free cereal, skimmed milk	Boiled or scrambled egg, slice of gluten-free bread
SNACK	Nectarine **(b)**	Orange **(b)**	Yoghurt	Apple and cheese	Banana **(b)**	Pear **(b)**	Melon
LUNCH	Chicken (small breast) salad with tomato and rice **(a)**	Homemade beef burger, coleslaw, potatoes **(a)**	Potato and spinach omelette **(b)**, salad	Homemade fishcakes with tomato salad **(b)**	Tuna salad, potatoes **(a)**	Broccoli **(b)** cheese chowder	Smoked salmon salad **(b)** with rice **(a)**
SNACK	Raw carrots	Apple	Orange	Nectarine	Yoghurt	Raspberries	Pineapple
DINNER	Beef **(c)**, rice and beans; melon **(b)**	Rice, prawn **(c)** curry, spinach; mango **(b)**	Sweet potato **(b)**, rice, bean curry; yoghurt	Brown rice, broccoli, chicken **(c)**, with prunes; apple **(b)**	Beef and vegetables Chinese-style with rice noodles; orange **(b)**	Roast **(c)** salmon, spinach and rice; homemade rice pudding	Steak **(c)**, vegetables, potatoes; strawberries **(b)**

Assessor report: The learner has created a nutritional plan for a teenager with coeliac disease.

Assessor report – overall

What is good about this assessment evidence?

The learner has used rice, potatoes and gluten-free bread and cereal to replace bread and pasta **(a)**. The learner has also included five fruits or vegetables a day to ensure a good supply of vitamins **(b)**. The diet is high in protein and minerals **(c)**, nutrients needed by growing teenagers.

What could be improved about this assessment evidence?

The learner has included only one nutritional plan for one individual instead of the two required. The learner should include the nutritional plan for the second individual to complete the evidence required for 2B.P4.

Quantities should be specified to ensure that Kaye gets the calories suggested in the introductory paragraph. There should be some indication of where the 2000 calories are allocated. Cheaper alternatives could be included where the family is on a tight budget.

(2B.M3) Compare nutritional plans for two individuals with different nutritional needs.

Assessor report: The command verb in the grading criteria is **compare**. In the learner's answer we would expect to see a comparison of the two different nutritional plans produced for 2B.P4.

Learner answer

Nutritional plan for Kaye, a teenager with coeliac disease

The plan shows a balanced diet high in protein, vitamins and minerals, avoiding gluten. Kaye likes fruit and vegetables and likes curry, therefore the plan has been devised around her preferences. She also requires a packed lunch during the week, therefore lunches consist of salads and food that can be prepared the night before. She has high energy needs, therefore a diet of around 2000 calories may be needed, mostly from potatoes, rice and gluten-free cereals.

	Mon	Tue	Wed	Thu	Fri	Sat	Sun
B'FAST	A fresh orange, cup of milk, slice of gluten-free bread	Skimmed milk, banana and small yoghurt	Gluten-free cereal, skimmed milk, banana	Gluten-free cereal, skimmed milk, grapefruit	Gluten-free cereal, skimmed milk, apple	Blueberries and gluten-free cereal, skimmed milk	Boiled or scrambled egg, slice of gluten-free bread
SNACK	Nectarine	Orange	yoghurt	Apple and cheese	Banana	Pear	melon
LUNCH	Chicken (small breast), salad with tomato and rice	Homemade beef burger, coleslaw, potatoes	Potato and spinach omelette, salad	Homemade fishcakes with tomato salad	Tuna salad, potatoes	Broccoli cheese chowder	Smoked salmon salad with rice
SNACK	Raw carrots	Apple	Orange	Nectarine	Yoghurt	Raspberries	Pineapple
DINNER	Beef, rice and beans; melon	Rice, prawn, curry, spinach; mango	Sweet potato, rice, bean curry; yoghurt	Brown rice, broccoli, chicken with prunes; apple	Beef and vegetables Chinese-style with rice noodles; orange	Roast salmon, spinach and rice; home-made rice pudding	Steak, vegetables, potatoes; strawberries

Nutritional plan for Mr Jones, a retired teacher with type 2 diabetes

Mr Jones likes trying new foods and he also likes cooking. He is less active and so does not need a lot of calories, but he does need a diet that enables him to control his blood sugar, has protein, vitamins and minerals. The diet has around 1200 calories.

	Mon	Tue	Wed	Thu	Fri	Sat	Sun
B'FAST	A smoothie made with yoghurt, berries and a banana, one slice of wholemeal toast	Boiled or scrambled egg, slice of wholemeal bread	Yoghurt, oats and cranberry muesli	Banana smoothie, slice of wholemeal bread	Skimmed milk, apple muesli	Blueberry smoothie, slice of wholemeal bread	Boiled or scrambled egg, slice of wholemeal bread
LUNCH	Fish fillet and salad with 2 crispbreads	Lentil soup, salad, 2 crispbreads	Pasta and bean soup, salad	Homemade fishcakes with tomato salad	Tuna salad, baked potato	Broccoli and cheese chowder	Smoked salmon salad with rice
SNACK	Apple	Apple	Orange	Nectarine	Yoghurt	Raspberries	Pineapple
DINNER	8oz Steak, rice and beans; strawberries	Turkey breast, broccoli, potatoes	Shrimp kebabs, rice, spinach; yoghurt	Baked potato broccoli, chicken; strawberries	Beef and vegetables Chinese-style with rice noodles; an orange	Roast salmon, spinach and rice; home-made rice pudding	Fish, vegetables, potatoes; strawberries

Both plans have a well-balanced diet and contain nutrients from each of the food groups. Both include protein in every meal as both individuals need a diet rich in protein and both include fruit and vegetables. Both plans include calcium for strong bones, and iron to prevent anaemia **(a)**.

They differ in that Kaye's diet is gluten-free, whereas Mr Jones has wholemeal bread and crispbreads **(b)**.

Assessor report: The learner has created two nutritional plans for two individuals of differing ages and with differing needs.

Assessor report – overall

What is good about this assessment evidence?

The learner has given specific suggestion for each plan and compared **(a)** and contrasted **(b)** the plans briefly.

What could be improved about this assessment evidence?

The comparison is very brief. Quantities should be specified to aid comparison. Kaye needs more calories. Mr Jones has type 2 diabetes and as such needs to manage his intake of carbohydrate carefully so that he can maintain his blood sugar levels at a safe level. It would be good to suggest the amount of potatoes or rice when they are on the plan. A wider range of carbohydrates such as pasta can also be included in Mr Jones's plan. Fruit such as apples can also provide carbohydrate so alternative fruits could be considered. Blueberries and raspberries are lowest in carbohydrate and can be grown at home. Including more of this information would give the learner scope to draw a more detailed comparison between the two plans. The contrast between differing energy needs of these two life stages should be drawn out.

Sample assignment brief 1: The effects of balanced and unbalanced diets on the health and wellbeing of individuals

PROGRAMME NAME	BTEC Level 2 First Award in Health and Social Care
ASSIGNMENT TITLE	The effects of balanced and unbalanced diets on the health and wellbeing of individuals
ASSESSMENT EVIDENCE	Written report

This assignment will assess the following learning aim and grading criteria:

Learning aim A: Explore the effects of balanced and unbalanced diets on the health and wellbeing of individuals

2A.P1 Describe the components of a balanced diet and their functions, sources and effects.

2A.P2 Describe the effects of an unbalanced diet on the health and wellbeing of individuals, giving examples of their causes.

2A.M1 Compare the effects of balanced and unbalanced diets on the health and wellbeing of two individuals.

2A.D1 Assess the long-term effects of a balanced and unbalanced diet on the health and wellbeing of individuals.

Scenario

As part of your voluntary work at a health centre you have been asked to present information to the service users about components of a balanced diet, its functions and its sources, and to explain and analyse the potential effects of healthy and unhealthy diets on service users, health and wellbeing.

Task 1

Describe – give details of – the components of a balanced diet.

Include the basic sources, function and effects of each of these essential nutrients:

- carbohydrates: simple (sugars), complex (starch and non-starch polysaccharides (fibre))
- proteins: animal and plant sources
- fats and oils: animal fats, vegetable oils, fish oils
- vitamins: A, B (complex), C, D, E and K
- minerals: calcium, iron, sodium
- water.

Describe sources using five food groups (meat, fish and meat and fish alternatives; fruit and vegetables; bread, other cereals and potatoes; milk and dairy foods; cakes and sweets).
Include the functions of food groups, e.g. growth, energy, maintaining body functions. You will also need to include Recommended Daily Intakes (RDIs).

Task 2

The effects of an unbalanced diet include malnutrition, vitamin deficiency, mineral deficiency and nutrient excess. Describe the effects of an unbalanced diet on the health and wellbeing of individuals. For each effect give an example of its cause.

Task 3

The effects of a balanced diet include raised immunity to infections, greater energy levels with increased concentration, and faster healing of skin, tissues and mucus membranes. The effects of an unbalanced diet are both short term and long term resulting from malnutrition, both over- and under-nutrition, vitamin and mineral deficiency, and nutrient excess.

(a) Compare the effects of a balanced and also an unbalanced diet for an individual.

(b) Compare the effects of a balanced and unbalanced diet for a different individual.

Task 4

Build on your work for Task 3 and include more detail for each individual on the long-term effects of having a balanced or an unbalanced diet.

Sample assignment brief 2: The specific nutritional needs and preferences of individuals

PROGRAMME NAME	BTEC Level 2 First Award in Health and Social Care
ASSIGNMENT TITLE	The specific nutritional needs and preferences of individuals
ASSESSMENT EVIDENCE	Nutritional plans and written report

This assignment will assess the following learning aim and grading criteria:

Learning aim B: Understand the specific nutritional needs and preferences of individuals

2B.P3 Describe the specific dietary needs of two individuals at different life stages.

2B.P4 Create a nutritional plan for two individuals with different specific nutritional needs.

2B.M2 Explain the factors influencing the dietary choices of two individuals with specific dietary needs at different life stages.

2B.M3 Compare nutritional plans for two individuals with different nutritional needs.

2B.D2 Discuss how factors influence the dietary choices of two individuals with specific dietary needs at different life stages.

Scenario

The practice nurse now asks you to create a nutritional plan for two people, outlining their specific needs and considering their different life stages and specific dietary needs.

The nurse has asked you to use two case studies based on different age groups and different health needs, for example, a teenager with coeliac disease and a retired person with type 2 diabetes. You will need to describe these individuals' specific dietary needs, and discuss factors influencing their dietary choices, such as cost, convenience, religion or personal preferences.

Task 1

Describe the specific dietary needs of two individuals. Choose case studies that link to diet (for example, people with allergies, a lactose intolerance, coeliac disease, diabetes, irritable bowel syndrome or Crohn's disease). Make sure you choose people from different life stages or you will not meet the criteria.

Task 2

Build on your work for Task 1 and explain the factors influencing the dietary choices of the same two individuals. These factors could include religion and culture, moral reasons, the environment, socio-economic factors, personal preferences, illness or underlying health conditions.

Task 3

The reason you had to choose case studies at two different life stages is so that you can now discuss differing dietary needs at different life stages. Discuss how factors influence the dietary choices of the two individuals with specific dietary needs at different life stages (for example, infancy, early childhood, adolescence, early to middle adulthood, later adulthood).

Task 4

Create a nutritional plan for each person and a short written commentary to accompany the plans. Considerations for nutritional planning should include factors influencing the diet of individuals and their associated dietary needs and the life stage of each individual and associated nutritional requirement, e.g. infancy, early childhood, adolescence, early and middle adulthood, later adulthood.

Task 5

Using your nutritional plan for each person, write a written report drawing out the similarities and the differences between the plans.

Assessment criteria

Level 2 Pass	Level 2 Merit	Level 2 Distinction
Learning aim A: Explore the effects of balanced and unbalanced diets on the health and wellbeing of individuals		
2A.P1 Describe the components of a balanced diet and their functions, sources and effects.	2A.M1 Compare the effects of balanced and unbalanced diets on the health and wellbeing of two individuals.	2A.D1 Assess the long-term effects of a balanced and unbalanced diet on the health and wellbeing of individuals.
2A.P2 Describe the effects of an unbalanced diet on the health and wellbeing of individuals, giving examples of their causes.		
Learning aim B: Understand the specific nutritional needs and preferences of individuals		
2B.P3 Describe the specific dietary needs of two individuals at different life stages.	2B.M2 Explain the factors influencing the dietary choices of two individuals with specific dietary needs at different life stages.	2B.D2 Discuss how factors influence the dietary choices of two individuals with specific dietary needs at different life stages.
2B.P4 Create a nutritional plan for two individuals with different specific nutritional needs.	2B.M3 Compare nutritional plans for two individuals with different nutritional needs.	

Knowledge recap answers

Learning aim A: Explore the effects of balanced and unbalanced diets on the health and wellbeing of individuals

1. Carbohydrates, proteins, fats and oils, vitamins, minerals.
2. Carbohydrates give energy; proteins build muscle; fats protect body organs such as the kidneys from damage; fats and oils also protect and help repair nerve cells and give some energy too; vitamins and minerals maintain body processes.
3. Vitamin A.
4. Vitamin K.
5. Iron.

Learning aim B: Understand the specific nutritional needs and preferences of individuals

1. Religion and culture, environment, socio-economic factors, family, class, peer pressure, the media, personal preferences, illness in general and underlying health conditions.
2. Dairy products.
3. After about six months.
4. Proteins and carbohydrates.
5. To help maintain bone density.

Index